Everything You Need to Know About

Measles and Rubella

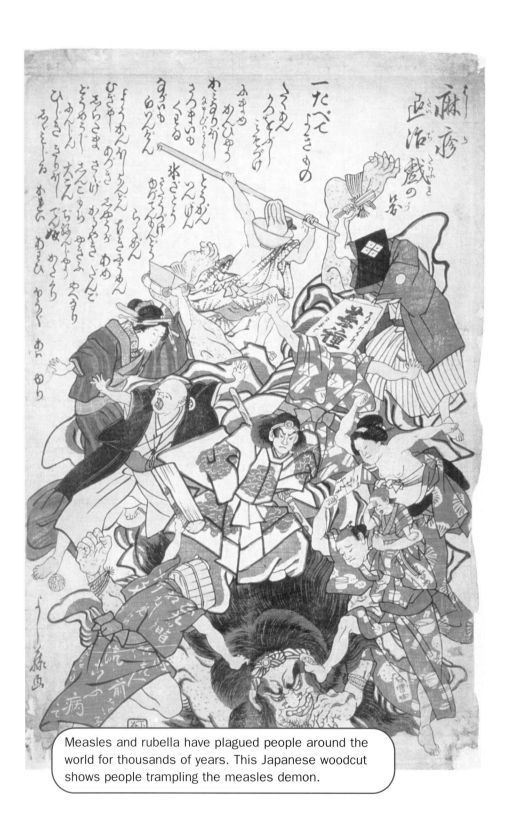

Measles and rubella have plagued people around the world for thousands of years. This Japanese woodcut shows people trampling the measles demon.

Everything You Need to Know About Measles and Rubella

Trisha Hawkins

The Rosen Publishing Group, Inc.
New York

For Elizabeth Duffy Hawkins

Published in 2001 by The Rosen Publishing Group, Inc.
29 East 21st Street, New York, NY 10010

Library of Congress Cataloging-in-Publication Data

Hawkins, Trisha.
    Everything you need to know about measles and rubella / by Trisha Hawkins.
— 1st ed.
        p. cm. — (The need to know library)
Includes bibliographical references (p.) and index.
        ISBN 0-8239-3322-9 (library binding)
  1. Measles—Juvenile literature. 2. Rubella—Juvenile literature. [1. Measles. 2.
Rubella. 3. Diseases.] I. Title. II. Series.
    RC168 .M4 H39 2000
    616.9'15—dc21

                                                        00-009721

Manufactured in the United States of America

Contents

	Introduction	**6**
Chapter One	**Understanding Measles**	**10**
Chapter Two	**Understanding Rubella**	**23**
Chapter Three	**Why Does Vaccination Work?**	**29**
Chapter Four	**Getting Your MMR Shots**	**39**
Chapter Five	**Measles, Rubella, and the People of the World**	**46**
	Glossary	**56**
	Where to Go for Help	**58**
	For Further Reading	**61**
	Index	**63**

Introduction

Measles and rubella are infectious diseases. Conditions such as heart disease and diabetes can be lifelong, chronic problems, but they cannot be passed from one person to another. You cannot "catch" heart disease or diabetes. But you can catch measles very easily if you haven't had your measles shots. It's one of the most highly contagious diseases in the world. Contagious, or infectious, means it can spread from person to person. Highly contagious means it can spread like wildfire. As recently as 1999, a million kids died of measles in countries around the world.

Measles and rubella are ancient. They have been making people sick every year in human history since around 2500 BC. Before that date, the homes of human beings were scattered over the countryside; after that date, people started living in towns and cities. They came into closer contact with each other. Closer contact brought more trade, more culture, more communication, and more services. But it also brought more infectious disease.

Sometimes a disease struck a whole community, and became an epidemic. When there's an epidemic, there is a chain of infection. The more people get it, the more chances the disease has to spread. If one person in a family gets it, then everyone in that family is at risk. If many families get sick, soon the whole town or country is infected. Throughout human history, there have been epidemics of infectious diseases, including measles, rubella, smallpox, polio, and, in our own day, AIDS.

Kids and young adults are the people who are most often infected by measles and rubella. A doctor who lived in Baghdad around AD 800 thought measles was a natural process kids went through, like losing baby teeth. He was wrong. Measles is not a natural process, it is a serious infectious disease. Measles can make you deaf; it can infect your brain; it can kill. Rubella is dangerous, too; it can infect a child in its mother's womb and cause it to be born with birth defects like mental retardation or blindness.

How does an infectious disease jump from one person to another? For many centuries, no one knew. Over the centuries, millions of children have been infected by disease and died before they had a chance to grow up. Today we know that many infectious diseases are caused by tiny germs called viruses. The viruses that cause measles and rubella are not the most dangerous germs that human beings can be exposed to, but they have been persistent, returning year after year to infect and sometimes to kill.

If you catch measles or rubella, there are no pills you can take or high-tech treatments that you can undergo. There are no cures for these diseases. But luckily there is a very effective way of preventing them. Prevention means that you do something, and because you did it, you won't get sick and you won't make other people sick. How can you prevent measles and rubella? Get vaccinated.

When a doctor or nurse vaccinates you, he or she gives you a shot, injecting vaccine into your body. Vaccination, immunization, getting your shots—they all mean the same thing. Given a choice, most people would say no thanks. Nobody likes to get a needle stuck in his or her arm or thigh. But vaccination works.

If you're reading this book in North America and were born after 1957, chances are you've never had measles. You've probably never had rubella either. You live in a time and place where most people get vaccinated against these two diseases as very young children, and today many people also get the now-required second measles shot. There is even a shot that vaccinates you against both diseases at once. It's called the MMR shot. MMR stands for measles, mumps (which is another infectious disease), and rubella.

Thanks to vaccination, measles and rubella are now quite rare in many countries. It's easy to forget how dangerous they can be. It's easy to take our good health for granted. But if kids stop getting vaccinated, the epidemics of measles and rubella will return. The measles and rubella viruses are not dead. They're just laying low.

Chapter One

Understanding Measles

If you're in good health and you get measles, you will probably be able to make a full recovery. But if your body is not strong enough to fight the disease and win, measles can be dangerous and even deadly. Before doctors and scientists discovered how to vaccinate kids against measles, everyone had to take their chances. You hoped you were strong enough to recover, but you could never be sure.

Measles Time Travel—If You Were You in 1962

Picture this: You're a kid living right there in your town, but it's 1962, and there's no such thing as a measles shot. Every two or three years, in your neighborhood, there's an outbreak of measles. It

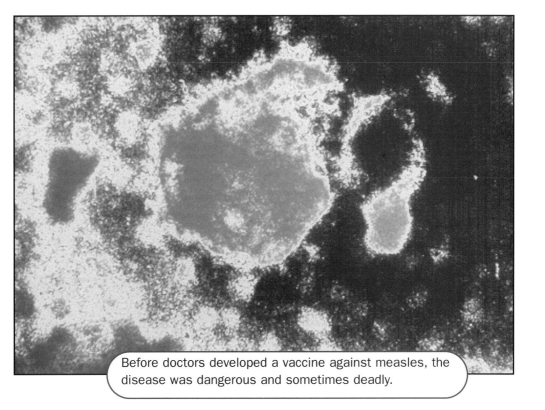

Before doctors developed a vaccine against measles, the disease was dangerous and sometimes deadly.

spreads from one person to another. Teenagers, younger kids, and babies become infected, and some adults, too.

Imagine you're the age you are right now. Some years, so many people get sick, they don't call it an outbreak, they call it an epidemic. It's 1962, and it's one of those years.

The cough might come first, or your eyes might get swollen and red. When you go outside, the light seems too bright. It hurts your eyes. The next day, you're sneezing, and when you blow your nose, you wind up wiping your eyes, too.

Your uncle calls and says that your cousin Gary is sick with measles. He thinks you may get it, too.

But the last time you saw Gary was a week ago. He was fine then, so he couldn't have infected you . . . could he?

The next morning you feel a little warm. You try to act normal but then you start to cough. Your mom feels your forehead and your dad puts a thermometer in your mouth. You've got a fever, it turns out. You tell your parents what your uncle said about Gary being sick, and your mom says there's no mystery anymore about what's wrong with you: You've caught measles from Gary.

Your dad takes you to your room and puts you to bed. He pulls down the shade on the window to protect you from the bright winter sun. "It's measles, all right," he says.

A day later you happen to notice a funny look- ing spot on the inside of your cheek. When you look closely, you realize that the inside of your mouth is covered with them. Another day goes by, and then the rash starts. First the red spots show up on your forehead and behind your ears. Then they start to spread down over your neck and shoulders. Your fever hits 105 degrees. The family doctor pays you a visit. There's no cure for measles, he tells you, you'll just have to wait it out.

You're in quarantine, isolated from the world. You're not allowed to see your friends because you're contagious, but it could be that you have

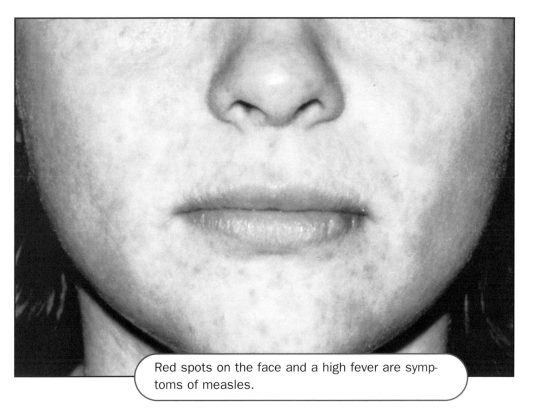

Red spots on the face and a high fever are symptoms of measles.

given it to them already. After all, Gary gave it to you and at the time he seemed perfectly healthy.

Your mom and dad take care of you, bringing you food and liquids and trying to keep your fever down. They've both already had measles, so they are immune—they can't get sick with measles a second time. But they forbid you to have any contact with your baby brother. They're still hoping that he won't catch it. They're hoping that you didn't infect him days ago, before you even knew you were sick.

The spots inside your mouth disappear. The fever finally goes away. You feel stronger. The red rash on your face and body gets dry and peels off.

You look out the window and you want to be out there more than anything, getting on with your life. But it's not time yet. The doctor says that you could still be contagious. You have to wait.

Finally it's over. Your body has won. You're fine. Good as new. You can't infect anyone now, you're not contagious anymore. You go downstairs and walk into the kitchen. Your dad is drinking a cup of coffee. He looks like he has been crying. You ask him what the matter is. Finally he tells you. Your mother is at the hospital; she has been there all night. They've been so afraid for your baby brother. They haven't wanted to worry you. The truth is, your brother is in the hospital, too. He's sick with measles and he is dying.

Viruses

In ancient Rome, a man named Varro had a hunch that diseases were caused by tiny creatures that flew from one person to another. The other people who lived in Rome at that time thought his theory was ridiculous. It wasn't until much later that scientists discovered the truth in Varro's hunch.

We live surrounded by countless tiny microorganisms. Luckily, most of these tiny germs are harmless to us, or even beneficial. But some of them cause infection and disease.

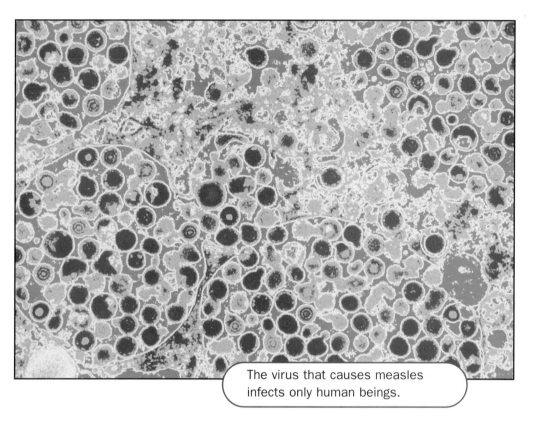

The virus that causes measles infects only human beings.

A Kind of Parasite

All germs are parasites—they live off other living things. They enter and infect a host. The host can be a plant, an animal, or a human being. Germs come in two varieties: (1) bacteria, which are living, single-celled animals and may cause disease, and (2) viruses.

Unlike bacteria, viruses are not animals. They're not plants either. They're in a class by themselves. They are not really alive at all until they enter a living thing, but once they get inside they can take over a host's body like pirates taking over a ship and run it to benefit themselves. Diseases that are caused by different kinds of viruses include measles, rubella, mumps, chicken pox, influenza (the flu), polio, and AIDS. Since we do not have

15

drugs that can cure diseases that are caused by viruses, we must try to use vaccination to prevent them from happening in the first place.

Like every other creature on Earth, viruses want to survive and reproduce. Some viruses first infect animals like rats, ticks, and mosquitoes and then move from there to infect humans. But the measles virus infects only human bodies, usually young bodies. No one knows where and when the chain of infection began, but measles has been living and reproducing inside human beings for thousands of years. No other home will do.

Actually, this is lucky. We can vaccinate all the kids in the world and hope to eventually destroy the measles and rubella viruses by depriving them of their only homes—it would be pretty hard to vaccinate all the ticks and mosquitoes!

Measles: An Acute Infection

Another lucky thing about measles is that you can get it only once. The common cold, which is also caused by a virus, can attack and make you sick over and over again. But measles is an acute infection. You catch it, it incubates in your body, it infects you, and then, if there are no complications, you recover.

These three stages usually take no longer than three weeks. And if you recover, then you can never get measles again: you will be immune. To survive, the virus that causes measles needs a good-sized human population—about 200,000 people—living in close contact with each other. That way it can move from one person to another more easily and always find fresh bodies to infect, year after year.

First You Have to Catch It

Before the virus can infect you, it has to get inside your body. When someone who has measles sneezes or coughs, little drops of moisture spray into the air, sprinkling the measles virus all around. If you happen to breathe in that air or come into contact with the droplets with your mouth or eyes, the virus gets a free ride into your body. Then you "catch" measles. When the measles virus moves into a community, it infects everyone it can. You can even catch the measles virus by walking into an empty room that someone with measles has just spent time in, if you come into contact with the saliva or other respiratory secretions that are still in the air.

Incubation

The symptoms, or outward signs, of measles don't show up until about nine or ten days after the measles virus first enters your body. This waiting period is called the incubation period.

During the incubation period, you may not even know you're sick, but the virus is attaching itself to cells in your respiratory tract and starting to invade

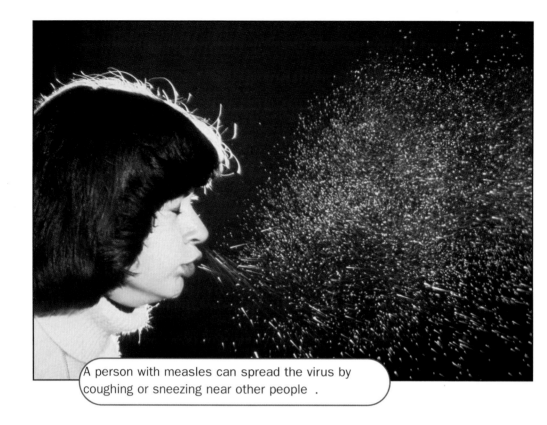

A person with measles can spread the virus by coughing or sneezing near other people .

them. Every part of your body is made of different types of cells. A virus can invade only cells that it can fit itself into, like a key into a lock. Unfortunately, many different kinds of human cells have receptors that the measles virus can fit into. That's why measles is so infectious.

Infection—the Battle Begins

When the virus gets inside a human cell, it uses its genetic makeup to take over the cell. The cell is forced to start helping the virus to make copies of itself. Soon there is an army of viruses. This army starts moving through the bloodstream, invading more and more human cells.

Meanwhile, the body starts to fight back. Special cells sound the alarm. They are part of the immune system. Different types of immune system cells fight the virus in different ways. Some of them start making cells called antibodies that are specifically matched up with the invading virus. For instance, in response to the measles virus, the immune system will start making measles antibodies. These specifically created antibodies will help the body fight the measles virus.

Symptoms—Now You Know You're Sick

Early symptoms are tiredness, a runny nose, red eyes, coughing, and a low fever. Then bluish white specks surrounded by bright red areas start to appear inside the mouth.

Two or three days later, you break out in a rash and the fever goes up to around 105 degrees Fahrenheit (40.6 degrees Celsius). The rash starts behind the ears and spreads downward. It is made up of flat red or brown blotches and raised bumps. It lasts for four to seven days. There may be diarrhea, vomiting, and stomach pain. The coughing and sneezing continue. This is the time when the infection can spread most easily to others.

While you're sick, one of the only things a doctor can do for you is to recommend a nonaspirin pain reliever to keep your fever down. (Aspirin is not recommended for an infection caused by a virus.)

Recovery—Now You Are Immune

The rash fades. The fever goes down. And after you have gotten well, some of the measles antibodies that your immune system has made remain in your blood-stream. They will stay there for many years, ready to protect you if the measles virus tries to attack again. Also, special "memory" cells in your immune system will remember this war with the measles virus and what exactly your immune system did to allow you to win it. The measles virus may try to make you sick again, but your body will be too smart. It will fight off the virus so easily that you won't even know it's happening. You will be immune to measles.

Complications—Sometimes It's Not So Easy

But remember, measles is an infectious, highly conta-gious disease. If you get sick, you may spread the dis-ease to those around you, and there is no cure for measles. The people you infect may be weak; their immune systems may not be as strong as yours. You are now immune—you are lucky. But they may be the unlucky ones for whom getting sick with measles means serious complications, lifelong problems, or even death.

Complications happen when the immune system is too busy fighting off the measles virus to notice that another disease is also attacking the body. With nothing to stop them, these other, secondary infections can be dangerous.

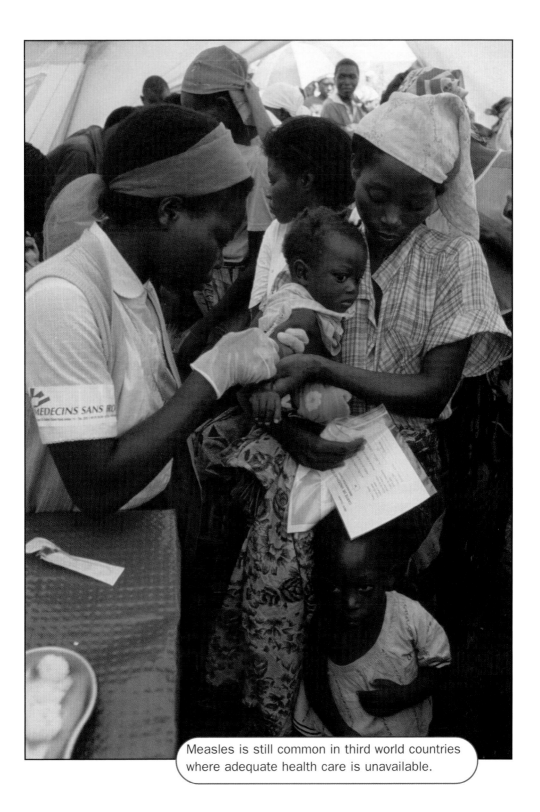

Measles is still common in third world countries where adequate health care is unavailable.

One of the most common complications of measles is pneumonia, an infection of the lungs. Sixty percent of the deaths that result from measles are from pneumonia.

Severe cough, diarrhea, and ear infections are other complications. Inflammation of the brain (encephalitis) occurs in less than 1 in 1,000 people, but 25 percent of those who do get it are left with brain damage.

SSPE (subacute sclerosing panencephalomyelitis) is yet another possible complication. It occurs years after a person is first infected by the virus. SSPE is a brain infection that starts with mental retardation and eventually leads to death. Mercifully, it is extremely rare.

Another danger is that if a woman who is pregnant catches measles, she may lose the baby or the baby may be born prematurely.

Death

One in 3,000 cases of measles ends in death, but in third world countries in Africa and elsewhere, measles is more common and the death rate is much higher. Kids in poorer countries have less money for vaccinations, health care, food, and shelter; and diseases like measles can infect them more easily and more dangerously.

Serious complications and death are most likely in children under the age of twelve months, children with weakened immune systems, and children who are starving or have a poor diet.

Chapter Two

Understanding Rubella

Rubella is sometimes called German measles. During the nineteenth century, a group of German doctors were the first to research the disease. But rubella is not measles. It is caused by the rubella virus. It is a separate disease and is dangerous for different reasons.

A healthy person usually recovers from rubella very quickly and may not even realize they are sick. But if a woman is infected with the rubella virus while she is in the first months of a pregnancy, the virus can infect the baby in her womb. Because of vaccination, rubella, like measles, is quite rare today. But outbreaks do occur.

Gina's Story

I live in Greece. In 1993, I married a boy who lived just down the street. I had known him all my life.

When we were seventeen we realized we loved each other. We got married and pretty soon I got pregnant. Everything went well until partway into the second month, when I got a little sick. I had a cold and a small rash on my face that lasted only a day. I didn't worry about it too much. But when I told the doctor at the clinic about it, he gave me a blood test right away, to check for rubella. He asked me if I had ever been vaccinated against rubella. I said no.

The test came back positive. What I had thought was a cold was the disease of rubella. The doctor told me that many people in Greece had become infected with rubella that year. And he gave me some news that frightened me. I had caught rubella in the second month of my pregnancy, and the doctor said there was a seven out of ten chance that my baby had been infected in my womb and would suffer from congenital rubella syndrome (CRS). A congenital disease is one that you are born with. If my daughter was born with CRS, she might be born blind, with cataracts covering her eyes; she might be born deaf; or she might develop bone disease or mental retardation. The doctor was very sad, but he suggested that I have an abortion. It was the best choice, under the circumstances, he said.

My husband and I stayed up fifty hours straight, making our decision. Finally we decided

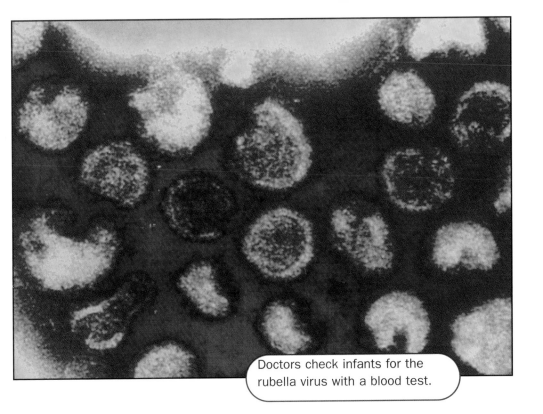

Doctors check infants for the rubella virus with a blood test.

I would go ahead with the pregnancy. During the next six months we prayed every night.

When I gave birth to our daughter, we felt blessed. The doctor examined her and tested her blood for the virus. He found no trace of rubella in her body. That's the only time I've ever seen my husband cry—he was crying with joy! We named our daughter Sofia. She has developed normally and is a smart, beautiful girl. And, of course, we have made sure that she has her vaccinations against rubella.

Greece learned its lesson from that epidemic of rubella. Now doctors in my country and all over the world know that all teenagers, especially *young girls at the beginning of their childbearing years, must be immunized against rubella. Many people get the rubella shot when they are a baby, but it is so important that young girls make sure they have been vaccinated. I tell everyone in my town, the best protection is to get the second rubella shot, too. If you've been vaccinated twice, you are sure to be immune. I was lucky in 1993, but other girls who were pregnant that year had babies with congenital rubella syndrome. Others had abortions. Whatever country you live in, learn from what happened to me!*

Rubella—Infection and Symptoms

You catch rubella the same way that you catch measles. Tiny droplets, which are released whenever someone who has the disease coughs or sneezes, carry the rubella virus from one human being to another. The rubella virus invades your body the same way the measles virus does. But rubella is not as contagious as measles, and living through it does not make you quite as miserable.

The first symptoms of rubella are like having a cold. There is a low fever. If and when the rash develops, it may last for one to five days. This rash is fine and pink, and spreads from the forehead and face downward. Some of the lymph nodes may become enlarged, especially

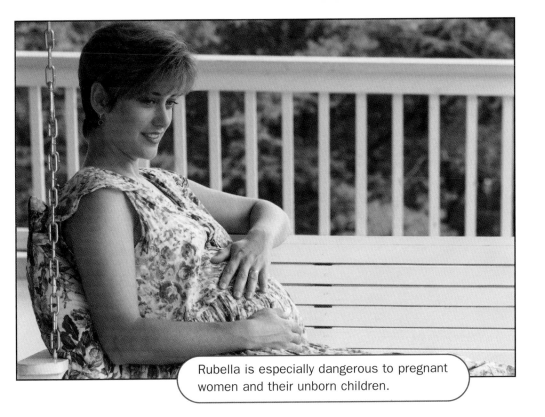

Rubella is especially dangerous to pregnant women and their unborn children.

behind the ears and on the back of the head. Teenage girls and adult women sometimes develop pain and swelling in the large joints of their bodies.

Rubella: A Danger to Pregnant Women

Rubella is a very serious threat if you are a pregnant woman. If a woman is infected with rubella while she is in the first trimester (first four months) of her pregnancy, she may miscarry, or the baby may be stillborn or born prematurely.

If the baby is born, it may have been infected with rubella while it was in its mother's womb. This is the most heartbreaking outcome of rubella: congenital rubella syndrome (CRS).

Congenital Rubella Syndrome

One out of every four babies whose mothers are infected with rubella during the first trimester of pregnancy is born with CRS. The earlier a woman is infected, the greater the risk to her child. A baby with this disease may suffer from many different kinds of birth defects, including mental retardation, cataracts, deafness, heart problems, or bone lesions. A child can die of CRS.

In 1941 an Australian doctor named Norman Gregg discovered that rubella causes congenital rubella syndrome. But it wasn't until 1969 that the rubella vaccine was licensed and made available in the United States. Today it is included in the MMR (measles, mumps, and rubella) shot. Protection against rubella is one more reason to make sure you have had your first and second MMR vaccinations, especially if you are female and in or approaching your childbearing years. If you're a girl age eleven or twelve or older, be especially sure you have had two doses of rubella vaccine. With high immunization levels—if enough people get vaccinated—the rubella virus will be stuck without enough human bodies to keep itself alive.

Chapter Three | Why Does Vaccination Work?

When you are vaccinated against a disease like measles, rubella, polio, or the flu, you become immune to that disease. Vaccination prevents you from getting sick. Vaccination saves lives around the world. Why is vaccination so effective? How does it work?

A Vaccine Stimulates Your Immune System

The substance that a doctor or nurse puts into the syringe and injects into your arm or thigh is called a vaccine. When the doctor presses on the plunger part of the syringe, it pushes the vaccine through the needle and into your body. The measles vaccine is made from the measles virus itself. The rubella vaccine is made from the rubella virus. Amazingly, the prevention for these diseases comes from the very viruses that cause the diseases in the first place!

The virus that infects you and makes you sick with measles or rubella is called a wild virus. It travels the world, and it is dangerous. But the virus that is used to make the measles or rubella vaccine is a weakened, or attenuated, form of the virus, and it is not wild; it is grown in a laboratory. Scientists have discovered how to grow a virus, weaken it, and turn it into a vaccine that is very safe and very effective.

When you receive your vaccination, this weakened form of the disease is injected into your body. The weakened virus in the measles vaccine will not make you sick, and it won't infect anyone around you. But it is strong enough to be recognized as a foreign substance by the cells of your immune system. The vaccine infects the body just enough to get the immune system to fight it. But because the virus in the vaccine is so weakened by its time in the laboratory, the immune system has a very easy time defeating it. After that you will have antibodies in your blood, and the "memory" cells of your immune system will know how to fight the virus if it ever attacks you again. Without having to go through the disease, you have become immune. If there is ever an outbreak of measles or rubella, your body will stop the chain of infection.

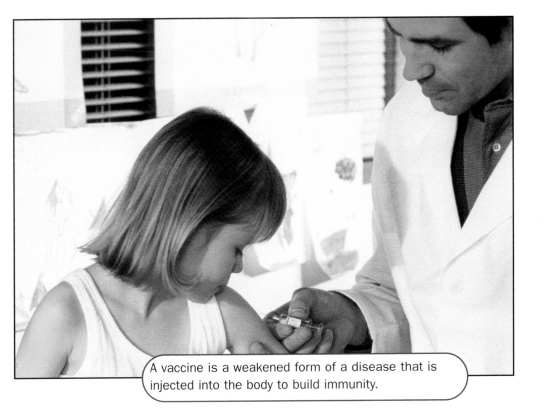

A vaccine is a weakened form of a disease that is injected into the body to build immunity.

Two Vaccinations Work Best

After one MMR vaccination, 95 out of 100 people will be immune to measles and rubella for the rest of their lives. After a second measles shot, 99 out of 100 people will become immune. Doing the math, that's a 4 percent improvement. Four percent may not seem like much of a difference, but if 4 people out of 100 are unprotected, then 4 out of 100 people can get measles or rubella and spread it to other people who are not yet immune. The MMR vaccination is good but not perfect. Once in a while it doesn't "take." Four infected people out of 100 can cause an outbreak of disease—that's why everyone should get two MMR shots.

Vaccination—Links to the Past

The idea of vaccination—injecting a weakened form of the virus that causes a disease into a person's body in order to make the person immune—is an unusual one. Today we know why vaccination works (see the previous pages), but early forms of vaccination existed long before modern science knew how to weaken viruses in a laboratory.

Smallpox

Throughout its history, measles has been linked to a viral disease that doesn't exist today—smallpox. The early symptoms sometimes made it difficult to tell whether you had been attacked by the smallpox virus or the measles virus. Both diseases were spread by armies, migrations of people, and traders.

But smallpox was far deadlier than measles. Even if you survived smallpox, you were left with pockmarks on your skin—you were scarred for life.

Variolation

In China in the first century AD, doctors were already trying to prevent smallpox. The method they used was called variolation: They took some of the scabs or pus from the skin of a person who was infected with smallpox and put it into the body of a healthy person who wanted to become immune and avoid getting the disease. Sometimes smallpox scabs were dried, made into a powder, and

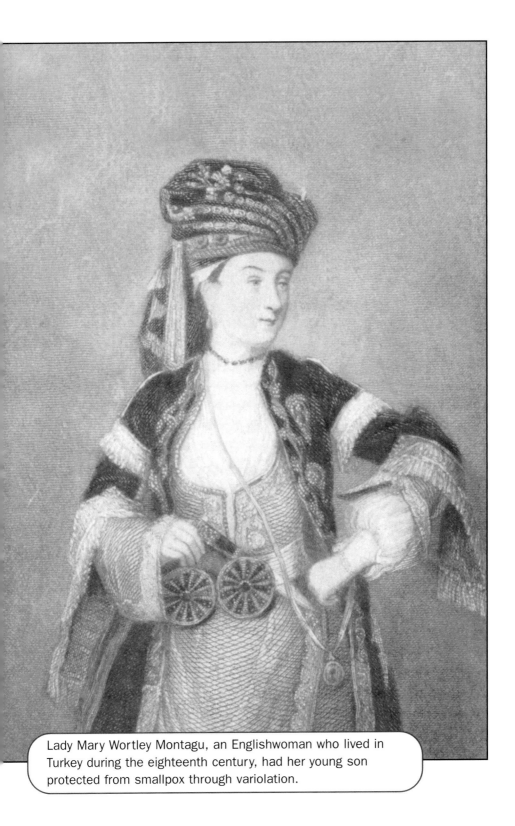

Lady Mary Wortley Montagu, an Englishwoman who lived in Turkey during the eighteenth century, had her young son protected from smallpox through variolation.

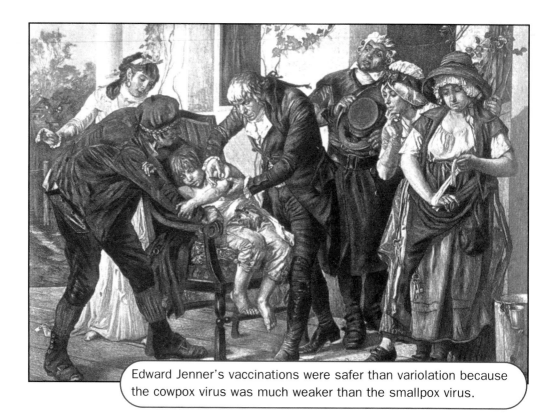

Edward Jenner's vaccinations were safer than variolation because the cowpox virus was much weaker than the smallpox virus.

inhaled through the nose. Sometimes the method was to remove the liquid from one person's smallpox sore and rub it into a cut or needle scratch on the arm of another. Variolation was practiced in India, Persia, and Turkey.

In 1718, Lady Mary Wortley Montagu, an Englishwoman who was living in Turkey, observed the variolation procedure. She had been infected with smallpox at twenty-six, and her face had been permanently scarred. She wanted to protect her six-year-old son from the disease. She had him variolated by Dr. Maitland, an Englishman who had learned how to do the procedure. Her chaplain was against it and told her it was un-Christian, but she went ahead with it anyway, and her son remained free of smallpox.

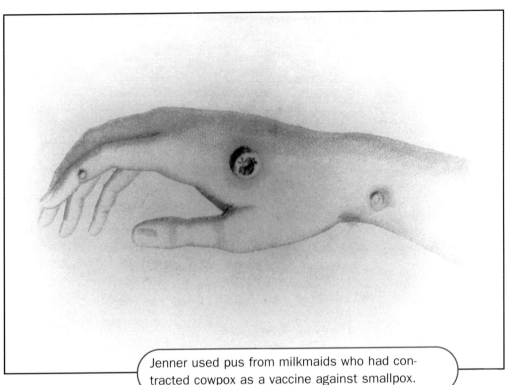

Jenner used pus from milkmaids who had contracted cowpox as a vaccine against smallpox.

Edward Jenner and Milkmaids

Variolation often worked, but it was risky. It involved cutting open the skin and putting a little bit of smallpox virus right into the bloodstream. It immunized many people, but other people got very sick and died. In 1798, Edward Jenner discovered a safer way. Jenner observed the smooth cheeks of milkmaids. He wondered why none of them seemed to have smallpox scars and pockmarks. He realized it was because they had been exposed to cowpox, a much less serious disease. The young women had caught cowpox from the cows they milked. When they recovered from cowpox, they became immune, and that immunity turned out to protect them against the dread disease of smallpox as well.

Jenner started using the pus from people who had cowpox to protect people against smallpox. The scientific name for cowpox virus is vaccinia. That's where we get the word "vaccination." Jenner's vaccinations were much safer than variolation, because the virus he used—cowpox—was much weaker than the smallpox virus.

Since Jenner's time, because of efforts all over the world to vaccinate people against it, smallpox has disappeared. There is no smallpox virus in the world today, except in a test tube, and hopefully even that bit of weakened virus will soon be thrown away. Smallpox is the only infectious disease that mankind has totally destroyed.

In 1977, the smallpox virus infected its last victim—there weren't any people left who were not immune. Because there is no longer any smallpox virus roaming earth, it is no longer necessary for people to be vaccinated against it.

Vaccination: For and Against

In 1798, many people were revolted by Jenner's vaccination method, even though it worked. They formed the Antivaccination Society. They argued that it was disgusting to infect a healthy person with material taken from a cow. They scoffed that soon all the vaccinated people would start turning into cows. Some were against vaccination because they said that it was not in the Bible.

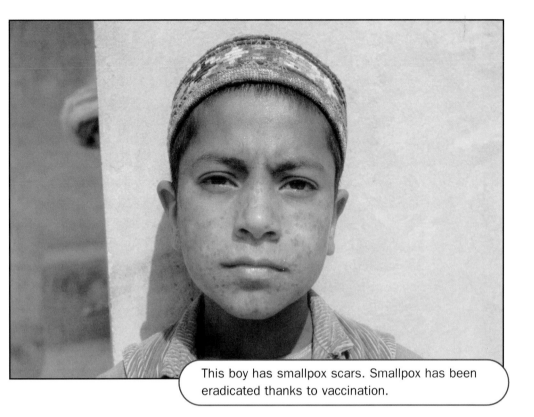

This boy has smallpox scars. Smallpox has been eradicated thanks to vaccination.

Even today, some people don't like the idea of vaccination—perhaps because they don't understand how it works together with the human immune system to protect people against infectious disease.

Measles and Rubella Vaccines Are Developed and Used

Even though Jenner had found a safe way to vaccinate people against smallpox, finding a safe vaccine against measles took time. In 1958, J. F. Enders developed a vaccine that used a dead measles virus. It was a first step, but the dead virus vaccine was not very effective and had some dangerous results. It is no longer used. In 1963, Enders found a way to make a vaccine that

37

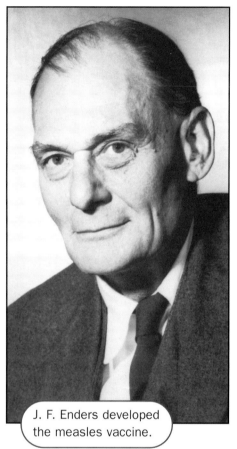

J. F. Enders developed the measles vaccine.

used a live measles virus that had been attenuated, or weakened, in a laboratory. This vaccine was very safe and effective. In 1965, the United States started a mass immunization program, trying to vaccinate all kids and young adults. In 1969, a vaccine for rubella was developed, and vaccination programs against rubella began. As a result of vaccination programs, there were only 100 cases of measles in the United States in 1997.

Chapter Four

Getting Your MMR Shots

Even though 95 percent of American children are now properly vaccinated against measles and rubella by the time they enter kindergarten, 5 percent, or one million preschool children, are not. And even though most eleven- and twelve-year-olds have already received the recommended two MMR shots, many have not. Visit your doctor or health clinic for a preventive check-up. Make sure you are fully vaccinated against measles and rubella.

Vaccine for Free

Because of lack of adequate health insurance, some families may not have a family doctor or regular health care provider and may skip their vaccinations because of cost considerations. As president of the United States from 1993 to the year 2001, Bill Clinton wanted to make sure that all the children in the country were able to receive the proper vaccinations, including their MMR shots. One program that was set up is the Vaccines for Children program, which provides free vaccines to doctors and clinics for their patients who need them.

Connecting with a Doctor or Health Care Provider

If you need to be connected to a doctor or health clinic so you can be given your vaccinations for free, there are toll-free information hotlines that can refer you to clinics in your local area. For information in English, call 1-800-232-2522. For information in Spanish, call 1-800-232-0233.

Recommended Vaccination Schedule

* **First MMR Shot.** Kids should get their first MMR shot between the ages of twelve and fifteen months. Getting it earlier than that won't work, because for the first year or so of life, babies inherit passive immunity from their mothers. As long as the baby is passively immune, the vaccine won't be able to stimulate the baby's immune system to produce its own antibodies. After the inherited passive immunity fades, then the first MMR shot should be given. Check with your doctor about the best time to vaccinate a young baby.

* **Second MMR Shot.** Kids usually get their second MMR shot when they are between four and six years old or when they turn eleven or

twelve. But these shots can be given at any age, as long as there is a period of time between the first and second.

◆ **Visiting Your Doctor and Keeping a Vaccination Record.** Your doctor or clinic can keep track of your medical history, including your vaccination records. Very young kids need to get a number of different shots in addition to the MMR vaccinations. Keeping a record is important, especially if you move or change health care providers. You will also need a record of your two MMR vaccinations because schools and some colleges will want to make sure that you have received your shots. Kids and young adults work and play in close contact with each other in schools and day-care centers, so diseases can spread easily. Most schools have a "no shots, no school" policy.

◆ **If You Are Unprotected.** If you have not been properly vaccinated and think that you have been exposed to someone who has measles or rubella, contact your doctor or your local health department immediately. It's possible that if you get vaccinated within a day or two, you will be able to protect yourself from the disease.

Sometimes doctors give shots of immunoglobulin to unvaccinated people who have been exposed to the measles or rubella virus. This is a shot that injects the antibodies directly into your body, but it is only a partial, short-term protection. It does not stimulate your immune system and teach your body how to protect itself and produce its own antibodies. Immunoglobulin gives you passive immunity to measles or rubella. But what you really need is the active immunity that the MMR vaccinations can provide.

Reportable Diseases

Measles and rubella are "reportable" diseases. A person who becomes infected by measles or rubella should report the illness to his or her doctor or health clinic, and doctors are required to report every case of measles or rubella they diagnose to the local health department. That way, all the doctors and health workers can be on the alert for other people who may be infected. To keep the disease from spreading, the local health department may decide to vaccinate certain groups of children and adults who live or work in the area.

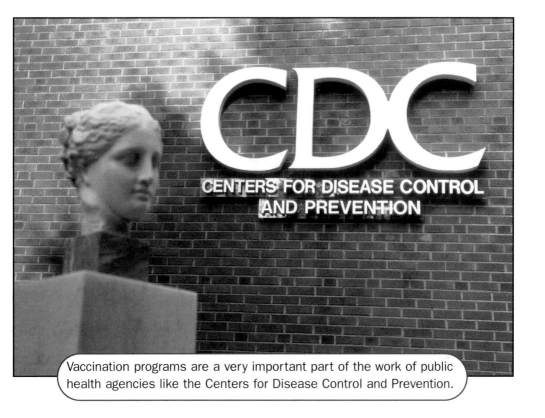

Vaccination programs are a very important part of the work of public health agencies like the Centers for Disease Control and Prevention.

If the disease has already spread, infected people of all ages can get prompt and correct diagnosis and medical supervision.

Public Health

There are governmental departments and agencies that work to improve people's health in your community, the country, and the world. Vaccination programs are a very important part of what they do. Every county, state, and province has a health department. There are also national public health agencies like the Centers for Disease Control and Prevention (CDC) in the United States, Health Canada in Canada, and international agencies like the World

Health Organization (WHO), which is sponsored by the United Nations.

For a Few Kids, Measles and Rubella Vaccinations Are Not Recommended

◆ **Postponing.** If you are fighting off another serious type of infection, you should put off getting your MMR shot until you have recovered. You don't want to overload your immune system. If you are pregnant, your doctor may tell you to wait. You can reschedule your vaccination for a later date.

◆ **Who Shouldn't Have the Shots at All?** For a very small number of kids, getting vaccinated against measles and rubella is not recommended. Some kids are born with very weak immune systems. They might not be able to fight off even the weakened forms of the viruses that are used in the vaccines. Those with the symptoms of AIDS should generally not get the shots (but those with HIV but no symptoms should be vaccinated). Kids who are undergoing some types of treatment for cancer and kids undergoing treatment with steroids or other drugs that can suppress the immune system should not get the MMR shots. These people must depend on the rest of us to get our shots and thus prevent the measles and rubella viruses from ever reaching them. This protection of the few by the many is called herd immunity.

Herd Immunity

When most people have been vaccinated, a society or country is said to have achieved herd immunity. Today in some countries the vaccination rate is so high that even if a few kids aren't healthy enough to get the shots, the measles virus probably won't infect them because it doesn't have a chain of people that it can use to get to them. Society is like a herd of animals, and the few who can't be vaccinated are unlikely to get sick because they are living in the midst of a herd of people who are immune. Of course, herd immunity isn't 100 percent effective. With people traveling all around the globe, you can't be sure that you won't meet up with someone who is infected with measles or with rubella. Don't use the idea of herd immunity as an excuse not to get your shots! You can't afford to be that selfish. If you are healthy enough to be vaccinated—just do it!

Chapter Five

Measles, Rubella, and the People of the World

The most interesting—and tragic—stories about measles and rubella recount how these diseases have attacked whole communities. When a large group of people is infected, it's called an epidemic. When the diseases flare up in small groups of people, it's called an outbreak.

The measles and rubella viruses depend on being able to spread from person to person, forming a chain of infection. By the time one person recovers, someone else is coming down with the disease. The virus is on the move, entering body after body. Today, every vaccinated and fully immunized person breaks that chain of infection. But without vaccination, epidemics can strike.

Examples of Measles Epidemics

Mexico

Almost 500 years ago, measles and other infections crossed the Atlantic Ocean for the first time and came to the Americas inside the bodies of the Spanish soldiers who invaded Mexico.

The native peoples who lived in Mexico had never had measles before, and if a group of people has never been exposed to a certain virus, it hits them much harder. Within fifty years, out of a population of 30 million, only 3 million of the Mexican people were left alive. The Spanish soldiers were cruel, but their measles killed far more people than their weapons did.

Fiji

In 1875, the chief of the Fiji Islands made a sea voyage to Australia to sign a treaty. When the chief and his followers sailed for home aboard an Australian ship, one of the chief's sons got sick with measles—though unknown in Fiji, measles was common in Australia. The Australian sailors knew how contagious measles could be, so the sick son was isolated from everyone else, or quarantined. The Australians built a little hut for him on the deck, and those among them who had already had measles and were immune brought him food and water. No one else was allowed near him. The quarantine seemed successful. It seemed as though none of the other people from Fiji who were on board became sick.

When the chief and his followers got home to Fiji, they prepared a great celebration in honor of the signing of the treaty. Suddenly, another of the chief's sons who had also been on the ship got very sick. Because they were so involved in preparing the celebration, they did not quarantine him. Soon other people were sick. And then more. Some died from the complications of measles, some starved to death—so many people were sick, there weren't enough healthy people to gather food, cook, and keep the society going. One out of four people—30,000 in all—died from the complications of measles.

Outbreaks in the United States, 1989–1991

Let's jump ahead to our own time. In the 1980s, the United States had a measles vaccination program and was aiming to completely eliminate measles from the country by the year 1990. But because more and more people were getting vaccinated and fewer and fewer people were getting sick, it seemed as though measles was no longer any real threat. People forgot. Doctors, parents, and public health workers began to take young people's health for granted.

The nation was shocked when measles made a come-back, infecting 55,000 young people, mostly in inner city neighborhoods and at colleges. Thousands were hospitalized, and 132 people, mostly kids, died.

In some of the areas where the measles outbreaks occurred, only 50 percent of two-year-olds had gotten their first measles shot. Most of the college students had been vaccinated as young children, but some of them still came down with measles—doctors learned the hard way that the first measles shot is effective only 95 percent of the time. And a 5 percent failure rate—which leaves 5 out of every 100 kids unprotected—is enough to give the measles virus enough unprotected bodies to attack and infect. At Siena College in Albany, New York, the basketball team wound up playing their championship game in an empty gym. Unlike the people of Fiji, Siena College officials realized that in a large crowd, the measles virus would be able to infect large numbers of people. The game went on, but no crowd was allowed in the gym.

Today—Who Is Getting Vaccinated?

Today, vaccination rates in the United States, Canada, and most of the other countries in the world are higher than ever before. The United State learned from the outbreaks of 1989–1991. Today the policy is: No shots, no school. We can still do better, but we are on the right track.

Today—Who Is Not Getting Vaccinated?

* **War and Famine.** In countries where there is war or famine, it is difficult for people to receive preventive health care, including vaccinations. Sometimes the measles vaccine is just not available. In countries like Iraq, which have been put under economic sanctions by other countries, many children do not get the vaccinations they need.

* **Religious Objections.** Some parents in the United States and other countries do not get their kids vaccinated because it goes against their religious beliefs. In the Netherlands, 1,750 cases of measles were reported from April 1999 to January 2000. Forty children were admitted to hospitals with serious complications including encephalitis, pneumonia, and ear and eye infections. Three children died. Ninety-nine percent of the sick kids had never been vaccinated against measles because their parents felt it was against their religion.

* **The Current MMR Vaccine Controversy.** In the United States and England, some parents whose children have become autistic believe that the condition may have been triggered by the MMR shot. Autism is a disorder that starts in infancy and causes an inability to interact

with others, repetitive behavior, and problems with language. But there is no medical evidence that autism can be caused by an MMR shot. Recent research shows that autism is caused by something in a child's genetic makeup. But some parents are still fearful. More studies will continue whenever fears about vaccination arise. It's important to make sure vaccinations are safe, and to make sure people know they are safe. If parents stop vaccinating their kids, measles and rubella will start up again.

Imported Measles

Most of the measles cases that have been reported in the United States in recent years have been "imported." Just as products made in other countries are imported into the United States to be sold to American customers, so the measles virus finds ways to enter the United States inside the bodies of travelers and visitors from foreign countries. For example, in 1994, a Rutgers University student caught measles while vacationing in Spain—after his return, the virus spread and infected twenty other students. The New Jersey Health Department declared a measles emergency. To keep the disease from spreading further, 22,000 Rutgers students, faculty, and staff were vaccinated at free immunization clinics. Today, almost every case of measles

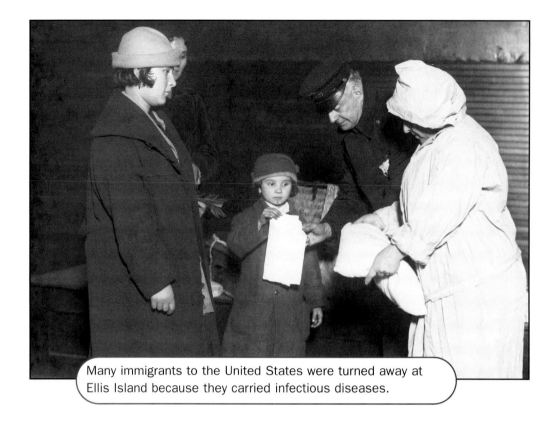

Many immigrants to the United States were turned away at Ellis Island because they carried infectious diseases.

and rubella in the United States is traced to someone who has come from or visited a foreign country.

Can You Build a Wall Around a Country?

It's hard to protect a country from disease by keeping foreigners out, but in the past, it has been tried.

Back in the 1300s, members of the government of Venice, Italy, stopped ships from landing in their harbor if they thought that the people on board had an infectious disease. The people who governed and lived in Venice were frightened; they were trying to protect the people of their city from disease.

At Ellis Island, in the New York harbor, where many immigrants came in the nineteenth and early twentieth centuries as they tried to enter the United States, many people were turned back because they were sick with infectious diseases.

This strategy of keeping a country healthy by keeping out foreigners who have or may have diseases doesn't work anymore, if it ever did. Today, international travel is so fast, there isn't a way to screen people for disease—they may have no symptoms when they enter the country, but later they may become ill and infect others. Dr. Samuel Katz, a pediatrician at Duke University, says that since vaccine-preventable diseases such as measles still occur worldwide, they are "not further than a jet ride away."

The Future—Getting the Vaccines to the People

Health care issues are inseparable from politics and economics. One of the most difficult problems is delivery—getting medications and vaccines to kids and adults who need them. Bill Gates, head of the Microsoft Corporation, has pledged $750 million to a fund to buy and distribute vaccines to developing countries. The group that will carry out this effort is called Global Alliance for Vaccines and Immunization (GAVI). GAVI is funded by governments and private foundations. When GAVI announced its new vaccination campaign, The Children's Challenge, in 1999, the organization said that getting more kids vaccinated could save three million lives a year.

Carol Bellamy of Unicef is hoping that GAVI will achieve its goal of making vaccinations available worldwide, but she admits that: "This is a crazy world we live in and . . . one of the problems we have is how many countries are at war and how we can get immunizations to the children in those areas."

Can Measles and Rubella Be Eradicated?

Health organizations have wanted to eradicate measles and rubella for a long time. But the viruses hang on. Eradication would mean that there would no longer be any measles or rubella viruses left alive. So far, smallpox is the only infectious disease that has been eradicated by mankind. Vaccination and careful reporting of individual cases of the disease are what did it. Some people think that measles and rubella can be destroyed, too. Others say that worldwide measles eradication is an impossible dream, and we should just give up. Still others are working hard to make the dream a reality.

Today we must face the facts: If we want to be healthier, everyone on the planet has to get healthier, too. Our sense of compassion makes us want to improve people's health all over our country and the world. And in addition, our own self-interest demands that we make everyone's health our business. We're all in this together, and we all need to get our shots. More and more, our community includes everyone on Earth.

E-mail from the Year 2010

Hi. I'm speaking to you from the year 2010.

I know all about viruses. In the past few years, there have been a lot of diseases in my city. Our scientists are working on developing new vaccines, but some viruses are so new, they're still a mystery.

But at least we don't have to worry about measles and rubella anymore. A year ago, WHO, the World Health Organization, announced that measles had been eradicated. Eradicated means that it's dead and it's not coming back. Just yesterday, the news said that rubella, too, has been destroyed.

I want to thank all of you kids who were young at the beginning of the twenty-first century. You got your measles and rubella shots, and you helped all the other people who were kids back then to get their shots, too. I guess the measles virus got tired of looking for people to infect—it just gave up and died!

Now, in 2010, kids don't need to get measles and rubella shots anymore because there are no measles or rubella viruses left alive. Yeah! One less needle!

I just had to thank you.

Diego

Glossary

acute   Having a sudden onset, sharp rise, and quick ending.

antibiotics   Medicine used to treat some bacterial infections and diseases.

antibodies   Proteins produced in the body as a reaction to an infectious disease. They help the body fight the disease and stay in the bloodstream for years afterward, ready to protect the body if the same disease should strike again.

attenuated   Made weak.

bacteria   Tiny creatures that cause infection and some diseases.

chronic   Long-lasting, constantly weakening.

contagious   Communicable, or spread, by contact.

epidemic   Outbreak of a disease that affects a large number of people within a population or community.

eradicate   To do away with something; to destroy something completely.

immune   Having resistance to and protection from a disease.

immune system   The bodily system that protects the body from foreign substances and disease.

immunization   The process of giving someone protection against a disease, usually by vaccination.

infectious   Capable of spreading from person to person.

injection   A shot.

microorganisms   Tiny creatures such as viruses and bacteria.

quarantine   To isolate from other people in order to prevent disease from spreading.

vaccinate   To administer a vaccine, usually by injection.

vaccine   Preparation that is given to prevent a disease. Usually given by injection.

viruses   Tiny creatures, smaller than bacteria, that may cause disease.

Where to Go for Help

In the United States
Centers for Disease Control and Prevention (CDC)
1600 Clifton Road
Atlanta, GA 30333
(404) 639-3311
Web site: http://www.cdc.gov/

Immunization Action Coalition
1573 Selby Avenue, Suite 234
St. Paul, MN 55104
(651) 647-9009
Web site: http://www.immunize.org/

National Institutes of Health (NIH)
Bethesda, MD 20892
Web site: http://www.nih.gov/

National Library of Medicine
8600 Rockville Pike
Bethesda, MD 20894
Web site: http://www.nlm.nih.gov/

World Health Organization (WHO)
2 United Nations Plaza, DC-2 Building
New York, NY 10017
(212) 963-4388
Web site: http://www.who.int/

In Canada

Canadian Immunization Awareness Program
Canadian Public Health Association
400-1565 Carling Avenue
Ottawa, ON K1Z 8R1
(613) 725-3769
Web site: http://www.ciap.cpha.ca/

Health Canada
Bureau of Infectious Diseases
Division of Immunization, Health Protection Branch
Tunney's Pasture
Ottawa, ON K1A 0L2
Postal Locator: 0603E1
Web site:
http://www.hc-sc.gc.ca/hpb/lcdc/bid/di/index.html

Web Sites

American Academy of Pediatrics
http://www.aap.org/family/parents/vaccine.htm

Children's Vaccine Initiative
http://www.vaccines.ch/vaccines-diseases/safety

Growing Healthy Canadians
http://www.growinghealthykids.com

Infectious Disease Society of America
http://www.idsociety.org/

Institute for Vaccine Safety
http://www.vaccinesafety.edu/

National Vaccine Information Center
http://www.909shot.com

VaccinesbyNet
http://www.vaccinesbynet.com/

For Further Reading

Bazin, Hervé. *The Eradication of Smallpox: Edward Jenner and the First and Only Eradication of a Human Infectious Disease*. San Diego, CA: Academic Press, 1999.

Benenson, Abram S., ed. *Control of Communicable Diseases Manual.* 16th edition. Washington, DC: American Public Health Association, 1995.

Biddle, Wayne. *A Field Guide to Germs.* New York: Henry Holt and Company, Inc., 1995.

DeSalle, Rob, ed. *Epidemic! The World of Infectious Disease* New York: New Press, 1999.

Humiston, Sharon G., and Cynthia Good. *Vaccinating Your Child Questions and Answers for the Concerned Parent*. Atlanta, GA: Peachtree Publishers Ltd., 2000

McNeill, William H. *Plagues and Peoples*. Garden City, NY: Anchor Press/Doubleday, 1976.

Mitchell, Violaine S., Nalini M. Philipose, and Jay P. Sanford, eds. *The Children's Vaccine Initiative: Achieving the Vision.* Washington, DC: National Academy Press, 1993.

Offit, Paul A., and Louis M. Bell. *Vaccines: What Every Parent Should Know.* New York: IDG Books Worldwide, 1999.

Radetsky, Peter. *The Invisible Invaders: The Story of the Emerging Age of Viruses.* Boston: Little, Brown and Company, 1991.

Silverstein, Alvin, et al., *Measles and Rubella.* Springfield, NJ: Enslow, 1997.

Index

A
acute infection, 16
antibodies, 19, 20, 30, 40, 42
Antivaccination Society, 36

C
Centers for Disease Control and
    Prevention (CDC), 43
chain of infection, 7, 16, 30, 46
Children's Challenge, 54
complications from measles, 20–22
congenital disease, 24
congenital rubella syndrome (CRS),
    24, 26, 28
cowpox, 35–36

E
Enders, J. F., 37–38
epidemic, 7, 9, 11, 25, 46, 47
eradication, 54, 55

G
German measles, 23
Global Alliance for Vaccines and
    Immunization (GAVI), 53–54
Gregg, Norman, 28

H
Health Canada, 43
herd immunity, 45
host, 15

I
immunoglobulin, 42
immune system, 19, 20, 30, 37, 44
immunization, 8, 28, 54
incubation period, 17
infectious diseases, 7, 8, 36, 52
    AIDS, 7, 15, 44
    common cold, 15, 16, 29
    mumps, 9, 15
    smallpox, 7, 32, 35, 36, 37, 54

J
Jenner, Edward, 34, 35–36, 37

M
mass immunization program, 38
measles, mumps, and rubella vac-
    cine (MMR), 8–9, 28, 31, 39, 40,
    41, 42, 44, 50
    and autism, 50, 51

O
outbreaks, 23, 30, 31, 46, 48, 49

P
passive immunity, 40, 42
pregnant women
    and measles, 22
    and rubella, 23–26, 27–28
    and vaccination, 44
prevention, 8
public health agencies, 43

Q
quarantine, 47, 48

R
receptors, 18
recommended vaccine schedule, 40
reportable diseases, 42

S
secondary infections, 20
symptoms of measles, 19
symptoms of rubella, 26–27

V
vaccination for free, 40
vaccine, 8, 29, 30, 37, 38, 40, 50
Vaccines for Children program, 40
variolation, 32, 34, 35, 36
Varro, 14

W
wild virus, 30
World Health Organization (WHO), 43, 55

About the Author

Trisha Hawkins is a writer and copy editor who lives in Brooklyn, New York. She is a graduate of Harvard College.

Photo Credits

Cover photos and pp. 11, 13, 15, 25 © Custom Medical Stock Photo; pp. 2, 33, 34, 35 courtesy of the National Library of Medicine; p. 18 © Lester V. Bergman/Corbis; p. 21 © Howard Davies/Corbis; p. 27 © Corbis; p. 31 © FPG International; p. 37 © Paul Almasy/Corbis; pp. 38, 52 © Bettmann/Corbis; p. 43 © Photo Researchers.

Layout

Laura Murawski

ML   6/01